TYPE 1

MW01296233

Smallest book
with Everything you need to know

Updated and Rewritten 2nd Edition

By
Dr. Shahriar Mostafa
MBBS, MPH

Preface

Now our lives have become busier than ever. Living in the age of information, We are connected all the time. There is so much to see, share, communicate and learn that we are always in short of time. Time has become the most valuable thing of our life.

On type 1 diabetes you will find thousand websites with million pages. You will also find many books with hundreds of pages. Virtually there is an ocean of information on T1DM. From this ocean of information what you really need to know is difficult to find. And its time consuming. So I tried to keep this book small. Here I have distilled the information most useful for the reader. I have gathered most of the updated and latest information on Type 1 diabetes. As it's a small book you can finish the book in an hour. In just 1 hour you will have all important information on Type 1 diabetes.

You do not have to read this book from cover to cover. You can start anywhere and slowly finish it. Use the table of contents to find the topic of your interest and start from there.

With knowledge on T1DM you will have the confidence, hope and information to live a normal happy life with Type 1 Diabetes. This could be a starting point for you to learn about T1DM, a starting point to know what you should ask your doctor and healthcare provider.

This is a good choice as a gift to your friends, coworkers or family who has Type 1 Diabetes, or recently diagnosed with Type 1 Diabetes. This gift will help them in their lifelong treatment of type 1 diabetes.

A point to note that this book mainly focuses on Type 1 Diabetes. For Type 2 or Gestational Diabetes there are other books written by me, available in Amazon. This is done to keep the book small in size and to keep the price as low as possible. Keep in mind that types of diabetes do not overlap each other. So one type of diabetic patient does not need information on other types for treatment, prevention or lifestyle decisions.

Acknowledgement

I like to thank following doctors for their contribution in this 2nd Edition of the book

- Dr. Shams Jaber MD
- Dr. K. Russel Hossain MD, CCD (Certified Diabetologist)
- Dr. Abdur Rashid MD, CCD (Certified Diabetologist)

I like to thank Dr. Talat Shama (Certified diabetologist). She achieved Gold Medal from BIRDEM for her work on Diabetes. Dr. Talat reviewed this book and given her valuable input. I like to thank her for giving her time reviewing 1st Edition of this book.

Dedication

I like to dedicate this book to Musfica Rahman (My wife, a pre diabetic), Samsul Huda (my father) and Samima Ferdousi (my mother, a diabetic). Thank you all for your support & coping with my hectic, busy lifestyle.

Table of Contents

Contents

Notes

Please remember, this book is not a prescription from doctor. Do not change, increase, start or skip any ongoing treatment without consulting your doctor.

Healthcare is ever changing, new data is added every year, new treatment emerges. This book will be updated every year. As you have purchased this book, I like to thank you and send you updated future editions free.

Please send me an email to dr.shahriar@doctor.com with "Type 1 Diabetes " in subject line, so I can send you future editions of the ebook completely free.

Please visit the following Facebook page and hit like. https://business.facebook.com/smallestbookonT1DM The Facebook page will give you latest updates on Diabetes.

You can also send email me at dr.shahriar@doctor.com . Feel free to email any question, suggestion or mistakes in the book. I will answer your questions and if needed correct my errors.

A review is very important for me. I can't reach others without your review. Without your review I can't identify and correct my mistakes. So I humbly request you, please write a review, even a small one (1 or 2 lines) if you dislike or Like this book. Thank you in advance for your valuable time.

Every effort has been made to make this book as complete and as accurate as possible. However, there may be mistakes both typographical and in content. Therefore, this text should be used only as a general guide and not as the ultimate source of information. Furthermore, this book contains information on Type 1 Diabetes only up to the printing date (January 2016).

Introduction

As soon as you learn that you or your child has type 1 diabetes you become terrified.

What happens in type 1 diabetes?

Why did it happen to me?

What to do to cure it?

How to control it?

How to explain this to a child?

What's causing it?

Thousand and thousand questions pop up in your mind. You search the internet which shows a million pages. You ask your health care personal but not satisfied with the answers. You become confused, afraid and angry.

But you don't have to be confused or afraid. You are not alone. Type 1 diabetes is a common disease. More than 350 million people worldwide have diabetes. With the popularity of the internet and social networking sites such as Facebook and Twitter you should not feel isolated at all. There are support groups for Type 1 Diabetes everywhere.

Keep in mind T1DM is easy to control. It does not keep you from anything the life has to offer. But you have to control type 1 diabetes all your life.

If your child has type 1 diabetes you have to prepare and teach him how to live with diabetes. He/she should know

- What is type 1 diabetes?
- What are the treatment options?
- How to give insulin?
- What diet is best for him?
- How much time he should exercise or play?
- How to check blood sugar?

- How to recognize symptoms and prevent complications?

Diabetes is like a shadow of you or your child. Like a shadow, it will always be with you. When controlled, like shadow you will forget even it is present. And in not so distant future, you or your child will be cured of type 1 diabetes.

Who should read this book and why?

This book gives you a complete picture on type 1 diabetes. If you are a parent of a child who has type 1 diabetes, then this book helps you to understand type 1 diabetes. You can explain your child about his disease. You will learn, how to help your child to live a happy and long life with type 1 diabetes. If you are a young adult, then from this book you will get all the important information. Knowledge is the key to win over type 1 diabetes, this book gives you that vital knowledge.

If you are a caregiver or a relative or a friend of a patient with type 1 diabetes. This book helps you to understand the disease.

I have tried to make this book easy & fun to read. The information provided here is medical information, learned from medical textbooks and journals. As it is information on a specific disease you may already know some of them, but reading them once again will help you refresh what you know. The book is written in question and answer format so that you can start anywhere on any question you like to know the answer.

Please Remember this book is not a prescription from a doctor. Do not change, increase, start or skip any treatment without consulting your doctor first.

Are Pharmaceutical companies hiding Cure for Type 1?

There is a common myth that pharma companies along with doctors are hiding the cure for T1DM. So they can make money.

This sounds silly, but people think there's a hidden agreement between doctors and pharma companies that the cure for T1DM, which has already been found, won't be made available so that doctors and drug and device companies can continue to profit from caring for patients with T1DM.

There's nothing further from the truth than this myth. Scientists are a highly competitive. None of them is holding back a T1DM cure because they can feel the others breathing down their necks! Thousands of hard-working doctors and other scientists have dedicated their lives to finding a cure for T1DM.

We are close to discover a cure but at the moment there is no cure for diabetes.

Emotional Issues and Self-Esteem.

Type 1 diabetes is a lifelong disease and has a major impact on your emotional health. There is continuous fear of complications. The special diets, medication, insulin injection and blood glucose monitoring is emotionally demanding.

Children with type 1 diabetes usually develop emotional issues. They tend to develop low self-esteem. The child feels as if he must be a bad person or have done something wrong to have been stuck with such a disease. The child may blame himself for the disease. Another negative effect of T1DM is you or your child may think diabetes damages your brain. The child may develop the idea that diabetes makes him less handsome or pretty than his friends. With all these you or your child may become depressed and it may progress to clinical depression.

Emotional issues should be treated by professional counselor along with support from family and friends. Professional counseling helps to gain self-esteem, reduce depression. Never hesitate to seek help form a professional counselor.

You need to understand diabetes is not your fault. Type 1 diabetes is an autoimmune condition.

Something goes wrong with our immune system and our immune system gets confused. It gets this idea that the very important islet cells in our pancreas that produce insulin are actually a virus or harmful to the body and it turns on them and kills them. We don't yet know exactly why this happen. But we do know that it has absolutely nothing to do with what we ate, where we live, what our habits are or whether anything happen to our mum during pregnancy when she was pregnant with us.

Another important thing to remember that people sometimes say really annoying things. You will find that everyone you meet now has someone who had diabetes and either had some amazing home remedy solution to cure it, or died of diabetes.

Just brace yourself, people get weird when they don't know what to say. They really want to show empathy and mean well. Don't get angry with comments of people, who doesn't have diabetes. Diabetes is the kind of thing you really can't understand unless you've got it. So be patient and listen with patience.

Celebrities with T1DM

Diabetes does not keep you away from success in your life. You need to believe that and explain it to your child. People with diabetes have won gold medals, play professional football, won Oscars and became Rock stars. People with type 1 diabetes traveled the farthest corner of the world, become millionaires and successful politicians. Following is a list of celebrities with diabetes, it shows if you control your diabetes there is no problem getting what you want in life.

"**Halle Berry** - Diabetes didn't stop her from appearing as the super-powered mutant Storm in the X-Men movies.

Nick Jonas - This 14 year old star of the pop rock band the Jonas Brothers was diagnosed with type 1 diabetes in 2007.

Adam Morrison - Diagnosed with type 1 diabetes at age 14, Adam worked hard and made it all the way to the NBA where he plays basketball for the Charlotte Bobcats.

Gary Hall - This Olympic athlete didn't let type 1 diabetes stop him from earning a gold medal in swimming.

Elliott Yamin - After being diagnosed with type 1 diabetes at age 16, he went on to become 1 of the top singers on American Idol in 2006.

Vanessa Williams - Not only was Vanessa the first African-American Miss America, she is also a diabetic.

Doug Burns - Mr. Universe doesn't let his type 1 diabetes stop him from being an award-winning bodybuilder.

Jackie Robinson - The first black baseball player in the major leagues had diabetes.

Anne Rice - The famous vampire novel writer is a diabetic.

George Lucas - The creator of the Star Wars saga is a very mild type 2 diabetic.

Chris Dudley - Before Adam Morrison, Chris Dudley played in the NBA with type 1 diabetes. **Bret Michaels** - The lead singer of Poison was diagnosed with type 1 diabetes at age six.

Bill and John Davidson - The big bosses at Harley Davidson Motorcycles are diabetic.

Mikhail Gorbachev - The former leader of the Soviet Union is a diabetic.

Johnny Cash - The famous country musician was a diabetic.

Elvis Presley - The former king of rock 'n roll had diabetes.

Sharon Stone - Halle's Cat woman co-star also suffers from type 1 diabetes.

Thomas Edison - The inventor of the light bulb was a diabetic.

HG Wells - The famed science-fiction author had diabetes.

Nicole Johnson - 1999's Miss America has diabetes.
Kendall Simmons - Busting heads on offense for the Pittsburgh Steelers keeps this diabetic athlete busy."

The list of Successful people or celebrities is a long one. Here I have given a small fraction. These success stories give your child confidence to deal with type 1 diabetes. These people show you that diabetes (when controlled) does not get in your way to success.

What is the worldwide condition of Type 1 diabetes?

"More than 350 million people worldwide have diabetes. A forecast from world health organization(WHO) Predicts this number likely to double or more in the next 20 years."

"In 2012, an estimated 1.5 million deaths caused by diabetes. More than 80% of diabetes deaths occur in low- and middle-income countries."
"In 2014 Diabetes worldwide estimated to be 9% among adults aged 18+ years".

"WHO projects that diabetes will be the 7th leading cause of death by the year 2030".

Type 1 diabetes mostly occurs in children and young adults. "5-10 percent of all diagnosed cases of diabetes are type 1 Diabetes. Type 1 accounts for almost all the cases in children under age 10. Seventy-five percent of all cases of type 1 diabetes are in individuals under 18 years of age."
Worldwide approximately 78,000 youth are diagnosed with type 1 diabetes annually. Incidence varies among countries: East Asians and American Indians have the lowest incidence rates (0.1–8 per 100,000/year) as compared with the Finnish who have the highest

rates (.64.2 per 100,000/year). In the U.S., the number of youth with type 1 diabetes was estimated to be a staggering 166,984. And the numbers are increasing.

Getting Type 1 diabetes when you're in your 20's, 30's, 40's or even 60's is more common than most people (including doctors and nurses) think. Type 1 diabetes was called Juvenile Diabetes for many years which was misleading. So if someone says you can't get Type 1 when older, they're wrong! 30% of people with Type 1 diabetes are diagnosed as adults.

What is Blood sugar or Blood Glucose?

As soon as you are diagnosed with Type 1 diabetes, your first question is "what is blood sugar? Where is it coming from?" It's coming from the food we eat. Food we eat is made up of protein, fat and carbohydrate along with vitamins, minerals, dietary fiber and water. All of these are important part of a healthy diet. After eating, food is broken down into a simple form of protein, fat and carbohydrate that our body can use. When food is broken into a simple form we get Glucose or Sugar from Carbohydrate (rice, pasta, bread etc.). Fat from oil, butter etc. Protein from meat, milk egg etc. The carbohydrate impacts most on blood glucose level. So for diabetes the carbohydrate or sugar part of our diet is most important.

About Carbohydrates

Most people who think of carbohydrate think of sugar, but there are many forms of carbohydrate. Followings are simple carbohydrates that can be digested by enzymes in the stomach and intestine:

Glucose - is the sugar that circulates in the bloodstream and provides energy for movement and for all the chemical reactions taking place in the body. It's a monosaccharide because it contains only one molecule of sugar.

Sucrose is another simple sugar. It is a disaccharide because it has two sugar molecules. You may know it as the sugar in sugar cane and beets or as simple table sugar.
Other disaccharides are lactose (milk sugar) and maltose (malt sugar).

Starches are carbohydrate made up of large numbers of sugar molecules.

Other types of carbohydrate are complex carbohydrates including **Cellulose** – it is the carbohydrate that forms the walls of plant cells; and fiber. These complex carbohydrates cannot be digested, which means that they provide no calorie and has no effect on blood sugar level.

The journey of carbohydrate within our body.
Carbohydrate starts its transformation from our mouth. Inside our gut food is mashed, mixed with enzymes and acid and broken down into simple sugar mainly as glucose. Glucose is the fuel used by our body to do everything we do and keep us alive. Sugar as glucose is absorbed in blood. Body delivers this glucose carried by blood to every cell of our body. It's amazing how blood supplies glucose to trillions of cells.

But glucose can't get inside most of the cells straight from blood. For glucose to get inside our cells we need insulin. Insulin works as a key for glucose to get inside the cells. In a non-diabetic person glucose from the blood gets into most cells when insulin is available to let it in. In the cell, glucose is converted into energy. If there's more than enough glucose to meet the energy needs of the individual, the excess glucose is stored in the liver and in muscle. When the liver and muscles are filled, additional glucose is converted to fat. Our body has an enormous ability to store fat, whether it comes from glucose or from other foods you eat.

INTERESTING FACT
Not every cell requires insulin to get glucose; some cells and organs take up glucose without using insulin. These include
The brain
Nerve fibers
Red blood cells
The retinas of the eyes
The kidneys &
Blood vessels

What is Diabetes?

Insulin is a hormone. It is made inside our body by an organ called pancreas and carried around the body in the bloodstream. Insulin works as a key for glucose to get inside the cells.
If pancreas could not make insulin. Or if your cells do not unlock its doors with insulin (insulin resistance) glucose stays in blood resulting increased glucose level in blood. This high glucose level in blood is called hyperglycemia. If this raised level of blood glucose continue all the time, then this is the condition we call Diabetes.

What is the difference between Type 1 & Type 2?

Although T1DM and T2DM share some of the same characteristics, they are not the same disease.

They differ in the following ways:
The cause of T1DM is a genetic tendency plus a virus. The cause of T2DM is heredity plus obesity plus a sedentary lifestyle.

Patients with T1DM have an absolute lack of insulin when the disease strikes. Patients with T2DM may have too much insulin when the disease strikes because T2DM patients have insulin resistance.

Most cases of T1DM occur in childhood. Most cases of T2DM occur after age 35.

T2DM can be controlled with diet and exercise alone. T1DM can't be controlled in that way.

T2DM can be prevented with lifestyle modification, T1DM is not preventable that way.

Diabetic ketoacidosis is often the first complaint in T1DM. It doesn't occur in patients with T2DM.

Most patients with T1DM are thin. Patients with T2DM are generally (but not always) fat.

T1DM and T2DM are similar in the following ways:
The clinical problem in both begins when the blood glucose rises too high.

High blood glucose acts as a toxin in both forms.

Complications of eye disease, kidney disease, nerve disease, and cardiovascular disease are similar for both type of diabetes.

What happens in type 1 diabetes?

Naturally the environment around us has vast numbers of microorganisms. Every second microorganism such as bacteria, virus, fungus etc. enters our body. Some of these microorganisms can make us sick. To prevent this our body has a natural defense mechanism. There are soldier cells to fight against bacteria, virus, and even cancer.

In type 1 diabetes our body's defense mechanism malfunction. Confused soldier cells attack and destroy insulin making cells called Beta cells of the pancreas. With damage, pancreas can't make insulin anymore. Without insulin glucose increases in blood. This condition where pancreas can't make insulin or makes tiny amount is called type 1 diabetes.

By definition, absolute deficiency or little and insufficient production of insulin by pancreatic beta cells leading to continuous hyperglycemia or high level of glucose in the blood is called type 1 diabetes.

Factors causing type 1 diabetes?

Many factors are responsible for causing type 1 diabetes. When a person has a specific genetic defect in chromosome 6. He has increased risk of type 1 diabetes. If you or your child has this abnormal gene, then you or your child has increased risk of getting type 1 diabetes.

With an abnormal gene, type 1 diabetes also needs a trigger event. A trigger event is usually a viral infection (with Coxsackie B Virus Enterovirus, German measles (rubella), Mumps or Rotavirus) or Exposure to an antigen such as Cows' milk.

To fight the trigger illness, our body starts to kill microorganisms using T Cells. Unfortunately, due to some defect sometimes these T Cells get confused. They think insulin producing beta cells of pancreas as some microorganism or Antigen. They start to kill these insulin-producing cells of the pancreas, leading to Type 1 diabetes. We still do not completely know what makes these T cells crazy. Scientists are working to discover the complete cause of Type 1 diabetes. We hope it will be discovered very soon.

On genetic predisposition, if a mother has type 1 diabetes the child has only 3 percent chance of getting type 1 diabetes. If only the father has it the child has about 6 percent chance of getting type 1 diabetes. But if both parents have type 1 the child has a 30 percent chance of getting type 1 diabetes.

Symptoms of Type 1 diabetes?

All other type of diabetes except Type 1 is almost always diagnosed by symptoms the patients feel followed by investigations. In case of type 1 the patient may be undiagnosed. Their first symptom could be loss of consciousness due to complication of diabetes. And as type 1 effects mostly children it's scary to say that they may not recognize symptoms or tell their parents about symptoms until they become acutely ill.

The assurance is, even if the patient becomes acutely sick or unconscious, don't panic. Treatment is available everywhere. With treatment patients recover completely from the acute condition.

There are some symptoms you may notice in case of T1DM;

Increased thirst - when blood glucose level is high. Our body tries to dilute the high blood glucose with water. To meet this increased water demand body signals our thirst center. So thirst increases.

Increased frequency of urination- In diabetes frequency of urination increases. Diabetic patients have high blood glucose. To lower this blood glucose, body tries to flush out the extra glucose through urine. That's why increased frequency of urination occurs. Diabetic patients may pass urine for more than 20 times a day. Waking up 3 or 4 time at night is a common symptom of T1DM.

Increased volume of urine - in hyperglycemia or high blood glucose. The body tries to remove all excessive glucose through urine. So the volume of urine increases up to 3 liters or more.

Other symptoms are
Weight loss, even after taking enough food.
Pain in abdomen.
Loss of appetite.
Nausea and vomiting.
Fatigue or tiredness
Blurring of vision
Mood change
Irritability

Patient may present with dehydration, unconsciousness due to the acute complication of T1DM. Recurrent episodes of urinary & genital tract infections are a subtle symptom of diabetes.

Lab tests for Type 1 Diabetes.

Besides symptoms, some tests are usually done to confirm Type 1 diabetes. Your doctor will decide which tests are needed. Some common tests for T1DM are;

Fasting blood glucose - Done after overnight fasting (No food or drinks for at least 8 hours). You have to give a small amount of blood early in the morning on an empty stomach.

If the test result shows fasting blood glucose level equal or more than 126 mg/dL (7.0 mmol/L). It is a positive sign of diabetes.

2 hours after 75g glucose - In this test after overnight fasting (No food or drinks for at least 8 hours). On an empty stomach, you have to drink 75g glucose dissolved in a glass of water. Then after 2 hours, a small amount of blood taken along with urine to measure the glucose level in blood and urine.

Blood glucose level equal or more than 200 mg/dL (11.1 mmol/L) two hours after 75g glucose. Is positive for Diabetes.

If you or your child shows symptoms of diabetes or complication your doctor may initially do a random blood glucose level, which can be done anytime. Random blood glucose equal or more than 200 mg/dL (11.1 mmol/L) is indicative of diabetes. It indicates that your doctor should do other tests to confirm diagnosis of Type 1 Diabetes.

HbA1c - Now a test called Hemoglobin A1c is the standard test to diagnose and follow up diabetes. It is an essential test. HbA1c measure glucose in red blood cells. It shows the average blood glucose level of last 2 to 3 months. It is also useful for treatment & follow up of a patient with Diabetes. This test can be done anytime. Empty stomach or just after food. Food has no effect on test result.

HbA1C level more than 6.5% is positive for diabetes. But if you have anemia, sickle cell anemia or thalassemia the test result can be false positive. The HbA1C test should be performed in a laboratory using a method that is NGSP certified and standardized to the DCCT assay. Your doctor will know and refer you to a certified laboratory.

SOME FACTS

For very young children, whose brain cells are still developing, it's advisable that the hemoglobin A1c be kept a little higher, up to 8 percent, until they've reached the age of 2. After 2 years of age low blood glucose levels will no longer damage their brains.

During puberty, as a result of the brain's increased production of growth hormone, it's extremely difficult to keep the hemoglobin A1c below 8 percent. Hemoglobin A1c upto 9 percent is the normal level for teenagers.

Other tests needed for type 1 diabetes?

To confirm and evaluate Type 1 diabetes doctors needs to do some tests. Your doctor may do following tests;

Autoimmune markers include islet cell autoantibodies.
Autoantibodies to insulin, autoantibodies to GAD (GAD65).
Autoantibodies to the tyrosine phosphatases IA-2 and IA-2b.
Autoantibodies to zinc transporter 8 (ZnT8).

Type 1 diabetic patients frequently have other associated diseases such as thyroid dysfunction, Celiac disease, Pernicious anemia, Addison's disease etc. To check other diseases. And to screen out the complications of type 1 diabetes following tests are done.

Complete Blood Count with Peripheral Blood Film
Serum ACTH level
Thyroid function test – to rule out thyroid dysfunction.
Fasting lipid profile – for vascular damage, heart diastase.
Liver function test.
Renal function test – to prevent of diabetic kidney disease (Diabetic Nephropathy).
Electrocardiogram (ECG) etc.

Other diseases with Type 1 Diabetes?

Malfunctioning defense mechanism that causes type 1 diabetes can also cause other diseases. Some autoimmune diseases associated with type 1 diabetes are thyroid disease, autoimmune gastritis, celiac disease, autoimmune hepatitis etc.

Thyroid gland – 7 to 30% of patients with type 1 diabetes gets thyroid disease. 25% of children with type 1 diabetes have thyroid disease. As our body's defense malfunction and destroy the insulin-producing cells it also destroys cells of the thyroid gland. Leading to hypothyroidism (low thyroid hormone). Sometimes hyperthyroidism (high level of thyroid hormone).

Hypothyroidism with type 1 diabetes increases the risk of hypoglycemia (low blood glucose). Your doctor will screen, thyroid auto antibodies (lab test using blood). It is predictive of thyroid dysfunction.

Celiac disease is a common associated disease with type 1 diabetes. In celiac disease cells of small intestine reacts to gluten. Celiac disease should be ruled out in symptomatic type 1 Diabetic patients. Symptoms of celiac disease are;

Abdominal pain

Recurrent loose motion

Erratic bowel habit

Weight loss, etc.

If you or your child has celiac disease associated with type 1 diabetes the diet plan is different. Gluten free diet will keep celiac disease patients' symptom free. Gluten is found in wheat, barley etc.

Monitoring of blood sugar at home.

Monitoring blood glucose level in blood is very important, especially for Type 1 diabetes. Getting pricked with Lancet 3 to 4 times every day is a painful process. But there is no better working alternative yet. You or your child cannot guess the blood glucose level without a test. Only if the blood glucose level is low a patient can feel it, but even then he can't feel how low it is.

For Type 1 diabetes you should check the blood glucose level at least 3 times every day. Before every meal. Once every week, check blood glucose 1 hour after meal.

And once in every two weeks check blood glucose in the middle of a night.

Lab test result for blood glucose is almost same using glucometer at home. Glucometer test result from the finger blood may vary only 10% of a lab test result. You must maintain a log with date, time, condition (empty stomach or after food) and blood glucose level. There are now apps available in iOS, android, and windows to easily maintain log of your diabetes.

INTERESTING FACT
Home testing of blood glucose was developed around 1980, it was the first huge advance in T1DM treatment. Before 1980, glucose testing was done with urine specimen, but this method didn't give accurate or helpful result because glucose generally doesn't enter the urine until the blood glucose is over 180 mg/dl.

By that standard, a patient with T1DM may never show glucose in the urine and still suffer complications of diabetes!

Benefit of Home monitoring of blood sugar?

Home testing of the blood glucose is truly a valuable tool that has made an enormous difference in the successful management of T1DM. Monitoring the blood glucose provides a snapshot of your or your child's metabolism at a given instant in time. It provides the critical information that allows you to choose the proper dose of insulin to keep the blood glucose in a range of 80 to 140 mg/dl. A patient with an average blood glucose in that range will never suffer from diabetic complications.

How much home testing for blood sugar should you do?

The more, the merrier, as they say. There's no doubt that a major difference between patients with T1DM who successfully manage their diabetes and those who have difficulty doing so is that the former test their blood sugar far more than the latter. It is recommended for testing at the following times:

Before meals to figure out the bolus of insulin to give for the meal, depending upon the current blood glucose and the amount of carbohydrates about to be eaten.

An hour after eating to gauge the rise in blood glucose with food and to respond with extra insulin before that meal next time

At bedtime to see if your child is going to sleep with a low blood glucose, in which case a bedtime snack is in order to prevent hypoglycemia.

Frequently check blood sugar when your child's sick because illness causes major changes in blood glucose.

Occasionally at other times just to see how a given food or a certain amount of exercise affects your child's blood glucose.

Steps to check blood sugar at home?

Start the task of home blood glucose monitoring with washing your hand using soap and water, again you will need to clean the finger with rubbing alcohol or alcohol pad before pricking for blood.

Now make the meter ready - Insert the strip in meter.

Prick finger to get a drop of blood. If blood does not come after finger prick by the Lancet, a gentle squeeze of the finger will help.

Place the blood on the strip, just touching the strip to the drop of blood will do the trick.

In few seconds, the meter will display current blood glucose level.

Do finger pricking on the side of the finger where pain sensation is low. If available, use low pain lancet. It will reduce pain almost to nil. Use alternate finger every time.
Carefully store glucometer strips. Only 2-hour exposure of strips to air will damage the strip. Blood glucose level from finger prick is better than blood from other sites (heel, ear lobe etc.)

Considering factors when choosing a meter

Here are some practical tips to consider when purchasing a glucose meter:

The meter companies may give away their meters. they want you to buy the test strips, which are different for each meter. Even within one manufacturer the test strips may differ for the different meters the company makes. The strips tend to cost about the same for each meter. If you find strips that cost significantly less per test, you may go with them.

Prefer a meter that has a data management program or app. You can add data to the program and the program will show statistics of your blood glucose level as visual table. Trying to determine trends in the blood glucose is next to impossible simply by looking at results in a logbook. The computer can do so much with the data. It will show you visually using charts your blood sugar trends. You can adjust your lifestyle and insulin dose on your blood sugar trends.

If your insurance company will only pay for one particular kind of meter or strips, you may have to go with that meter. But if you and your doctor are willing to go through the hassle of contacting the insurance company and requesting authorization, you may be able to use the meter of your choice.

Buy an easy to use meter. If you want your child to learn to test himself, make sure the meter is easy to use so that he can use the meter.

What is continuous glucose monitor?

Thanks to advances in technology, now we can use continuous glucose monitors (CGMs). CGMs obtain glucose readings from a needle placed under the skin. CGMs are worn on the body, similar to an insulin pump. It measures and display continuously whether the glucose level in the body is rising, falling or steady. CGMs are useful tools that complement but do not replace blood glucose meters. Because a CGM measures blood glucose from the fluid between cells, rather than from capillary blood, there is a slight lag time for results. It is therefore safest to rely on a finger prick reading when making important decisions.

The costs of CGM technology are high for most of the people. There are efforts to lower the cost. CGMs will gradually become more common and important tools for the management of type 1 diabetes, particularly for those who use an insulin pump.

Apps for record keeping of type 1 diabetes?

Monitoring and keeping the record of type 1 Diabetes is easy now. There are many apps for iPhone, iPad, Android and Windows. To give you an initial idea of these I have reviewed two apps. You can use these apps or find one of your choice.

Diabetes: M

Designed for smartphones and tablets this application is intended to help diabetics to manage better their diabetes and keep it under control. Users can log their values in this diary and keep the records with them all the time. The application tracks almost all aspects of the diabetes treatment and provides detailed reports, charts, and statistics to share via the email with the supervising physician. It provides various tools to the diabetics, so they can find the trends in blood glucose levels and allows users to calculate normal and prolonged insulin boluses using it's highly effective, top-notch bolus calculator.

"Diabetes: M" can analyze the values from the imported data from various glucometers and insulin pumps via the exported files from their respective diabetes management software systems.

Supports Android Wear smartwatches. The app is available in Android play store and iTunes store.

mySugr Diabetes Logbook

mySugr Logbook app is a charming diabetes tracker for blood glucose, bolus, basal, food, carbs, meds, pills, weight, a1c and more. It makes your diary useful in everyday life with playful elements and immediate feedback through your diabetes monster! Get motivated and involved in your diabetes therapy, today!

— No. 1 diabetes logbook app in 6 countries

— Most popular diabetes logbook app in the world based on five-star reviews and ratings

— Winner of Germany's "Focus Diabetes" 'Best Apps for People with Diabetes' award

Our motto: We make diabetes suck less!

FEATURES/ADD-ONS:

• Designed for type 1 & type 2 diabetes

• Quick and easy logging (meals, meds, BG's, and more)

• Personalized logging screen (add, remove, and reorder fields)

• Estimated HbA1c - so there are no nastier surprises

• CGM data integration via CSV import

• Daily, weekly, monthly analysis (and more)

• Exciting challenges for personal therapy goals

You can visit the iTunes store or google play store, there are a lot of apps for diabetes. You can download those apps and decide which app works for you.

Treatment options for Type 1 Diabetes?

Type 1 diabetes does not respond to oral medicine.

In type 1 diabetes our body does not make insulin so insulin is given from outside. If insulin is taken by mouth, it gets digested and becomes inactive in our stomach, so insulin have to be given as injection. The injection is given under the skin. If we give insulin in vein or muscle it works fast but works for a very short time. That's why insulin is given under skin. From under skin It's absorbed slowly and work for a long time.

Patient can take insulin by insulin pen, insulin pump or insulin injection.

Most of the people with T1DM needs a long acting basal insulin and a mealtime short acting bolus insulin. Insulin is not like taking a pill each day. You'll learn how to change the doses. Sometimes every day or every hour insulin dose needs to be calculated for different glucose level and other conditions. Pretty soon you'll start to get the hang of balancing your insulin dose with how you eat, drink and play.

Goals of Type 1 Diabetes Treatment.

When you want to control your or your child's blood sugar for a healthy and active life, you have to set certain goals. These goals will show your effort. According to these goals you can modify your lifestyle and treatment plan.

- Target Fasting blood glucose could be 6mmol/l and 2 hours after meal 8 mmol/l
- Your Target HbA1c level should be less than 7%.
- Target blood pressure is under 140 / 80 and Target LDL level is below 100.
- Target blood cholesterol is 4 mmol/L and Tryglicaroid 1.7 mmol/L.

Insulin, what are the types of insulin?

Since its discovery in 1921. Insulin has become the most prescribed drug in history.

As a drug Insulin is made from animals (cow, pig etc.) or Bacteria genetically engineered to make insulin same as human insulin. Some manufactured insulin is modified to work better. Those modified insulins are called an insulin analog.

There are many types of insulin.

Rapid Acting Insulin as the name implies, this type of insulin works within 15 min of injection and works up to 4 hours.

Short-acting insulin or regular insulin starts working in 30 minutes. It continues work up to 6 hours.

Intermediate-acting Insulin - It gets into blood in 2 hours. And works up to 18 hours.

Long-acting insulin reaches blood in 3 or 4 hours after injection. And works up to 24 hours.

There is mixed insulin containing rapid acting insulin analog and medium or long acting insulin. Given before meals. They start to work in 2 hours after injection.

What type of insulin you or your child need?

The type of insulin you or your child need must be advised by your doctor. It can be harmful if insulin is given in vein or muscle or in large dose. Never change your treatment plan without consulting your doctor or health care professional.

In general, most people with type 1 diabetes needs multiple doses of insulin injection or continuous insulin infusion.

To reduce the chance of hypoglycemia, insulin analogs should be used.

Insulin Dose Explained

The objective of injectable insulin is to duplicate the secretion of insulin by normal pancreas. Normal insulin secretion from pancreas has two parts:

Basal insulin - usually from a normal functioning pancreas, a small amount of insulin called the basal secretion of insulin circulates in the blood at all times. This can be duplicated in a patient with type 1 diabetes by taking long-acting insulin. The other way of getting small amount of insulin continuously is with an insulin pump.

Basal insulin deals with the glucose produced by your liver. If you skip a meal, your basal insulin alone should be able to keep your blood glucose levels stable.

Bolus insulin- normally the pancreas secretes a larger amount of insulin at the time of meals, called the bolus secretion. This amount is duplicated by taking rapid acting insulin just before the meal or regular insulin 30 minutes before meals.

While basal insulin influences your blood glucose levels in between meals, it's the bolus (fast-acting) insulin that deals with the carbohydrate contained in any food and drink you have.

Your doctor will determine the dose of insulin consisting of a basal dose and a bolus dose. Usually insulin dose is calculated by Patients weight in kilogram and multiplied by 0.3.

The first time a patient takes insulin, the dosage is based upon a calculated total daily dose. Your doctor will make this decision on dose,

Doctors usually follow these steps to calculate insulin dose:
Multiply the weight of the patient in kilograms by 0.3. (for example if a patients' weight is 40 kg, insulin needed (40 multiplied by 0.3) 12 unit per day.

Divide the total daily dose into basal and bolus dose by simply dividing it in half. (for example if patient needs 12 unit per day he should get 6-unit basal dose and 6-unit bolus dose.

The basal dose is taken once or sometimes split into two times a day, usually in the morning (two third of the full dose) and/or (remaining 1 third) at bedtime. It is best to divide the basal dose into a large number of units in the morning and a few units at bedtime.

Factors influencing the bolus dose of Insulin.

Your doctor will decide how much insulin you or your child need. Bolus dose of insulin is calculated using three major factors.

The level of the blood glucose before a meal – if before meal blood glucose is high you need to add two unit of insulin with your regular dose. If the premeal blood glucose is lower than ideal, you need to decrease two unit of insulin from your regular dose.

The amount of carbohydrate in your meal – generally for every 15 grams of carbohydrate 1-unit insulin is added. But the amount of adjustment varies with different people at different ages.

<u>Whether exercise has been or is about to be done</u> - Exercise generally lowers the blood glucose. But sometime exercise may increase blood glucose. Try to maintain a blood glucose of about 150 mg/dl during exercise. Take glucose in the form of three to four glucose tablets if the blood glucose falls below 100 mg/dl. Take rapid-acting insulin and wait before exercise if the blood glucose is over 300 mg/dl. Take half the usual dose before a meal before exercise if the blood glucose is satisfactory.

Try to exercise around the same time every day.

How to keep and store insulin?

Keep the insulin you are currently using at room temperature in a cool, dry place and away from direct light. Its best to keep regular use insulin under 30 C. Cold insulin injection is painful. If you keep your regular use insulin in a fridge be sure to take out insulin from fridge 30 minutes before using it. Keep it at room temperature for 30 min before giving injection.

If you need to store insulin for long periods keep it at 4 to 6-degree temperature.

Don't place insulin in, or close to, the freezer compartment.

Never heat insulin or keep it beside the source of heat (oven, TV, locked car, radiator etc.)

For travel, use a special cold bag or use a flask.

Check the expiration date and color of insulin. If there is clamps or the color changed do not use it.

Don't use insulin if:

Clear insulin has turned cloudy or changed color

The expiration date has been reached

Insulin has been frozen solid or exposed to high temperatures

Lumps or flakes can be seen inside the vial.
The vial has been opened for more than 28 days.

Where to inject insulin?

Insulin is given just under the skin for longer effect. And most of the time it's self-administered. It's easy to give insulin injection in your belly, back and thighs. Remember not to give insulin at the same site regularly. Rotate the sites every time.

Features of syringes and needles?

You and your child need to know how to measure and deliver insulin with a syringe and needle. It is the oldest and still most common method for delivering insulin. Numerous different brands of syringes and needles are available.

Common features of syringes and needle:

Syringes come in sizes of 1 ml (100 units), 0.5 ml (50 units), and 0.3 ml (30 units). Disposable syringes may be reused as long as the needle remains sharp and only one person use it.

If you're using less than 30 units of insulin for all shots, the 0.3 ml syringe is easiest to use. If you use more than 30 but less than 50 units, the 0.5 ml syringe is best. For more than 50 unit use 1ml syringe.

Needle size is either 1/2 inch or 5/16-inch long. Children usually use the shorter needle.

Needle gauge or thickness is 28, 29, 30, or 31. The higher the number, the thinner the needle. The thinner needles are less painful and are preferred for children and adults alike.

Steps to give an insulin injection?

For type 1 diabetes, insulin injection is the treatment. Your doctor will calculate how much insulin needed (Dose). Your doctor will also tell you how many times insulins is needed and type of insulin needed.

Follow these steps to give an insulin injection
Wash your hand with soap and water.
Check the insulin bottle for expiration date.
Check the insulin bottle for clamps, color change. If there is clamps or color change do not give insulin from that vial.
Wipe the cap of insulin bottle with an alcohol pad.
Clean skin where you will get the injection with alcohol pad or soap and water.
Pinch skin and fat with thumb.
Push the needle into your skin: With your other hand, hold the syringe at a 45-degree angle. Make sure the needle is all the way into the skin.
Let go of the pinched tissue before you inject the insulin
Inject the insulin: Press the plunger with your thumb.
Use slow and steady push until the insulin is gone.
Wait 5 to 10 seconds.
Pull out the needle at the same angle you put it in. Press your injection site with cotton for a few seconds. Disposable syringes may be reused as long as the needle remains sharp and only one person use it. But It is best to use Insulin syringes only once. Throw away used needles and syringes in a hard container so that the needles cannot stick through. Close the container with a screw-on cap. Keep the container out of reach of children and pets.

How to decrease pain when giving insulin?

The most annoying thing of T1DM is getting injection multiple times every day. It's a painful process. You may decrease the pain following these advices;

Inject insulin at room temperature. If insulin is stored in the fridge, remove it 30 minutes before you inject it. Cold insulin injection is painful.

Remove all air bubbles from the syringe before the injection.

If you clean your skin with an alcohol pad, wait until it has dried before you inject insulin.

Relax the muscles at injection site.

Avoid changing direction of the needle during insertion or removal.

It is best not to reuse disposable needles. Because needles get blunt and cause pain.

Try numbing the area of injection by use of an ice cube. Keep the ice cube pressed to skin for 2 minutes just before injection.

Always use a different site to give the injection.

When to let your child to take insulin himself?

You may want to delay the time until your child can calculates his own insulin dosage. Do not give the child to get injection on his own until you're certain he can do it properly.

Teach him to administer the insulin. Show your child how to take Insulin injection.

Tell your child that Insulin injection is even less painful than finger sticking for the blood glucose.

Teaching how to give insulin injection should be done early, around age 10 of your child.

When your child has sufficient hand-eye coordination, he must learn to take the correct dose of insulin into the syringe and inject it under his skin properly.

Keep up the positive reinforcement with praise, and minimize your response to mistakes if they aren't serious.

What is insulin pump?

An insulin pump is a small device. It gives insulin according to your need. From Insulin Pump insulin is given through a small, flexible, plastic pipe or cannula inserted in your body. The cannula or pipe is changed every 3 to 4 days. Insulin pumps stops the need of injection every day, saves you the pain.

The main advantages of using an Insulin pump are:
- A pump delivers a continuous, pre-set (basal) dose of insulin throughout the day and the rate of delivery can be customized to meet your needs.
- Dose can be adjusted to a lower rate late at night to avoid hypos and a higher rate in the early morning to overcome the dawn phenomenon (a well-known occurrence when sugars rise with the sun).
- Only rapid-acting insulin is used so it simulates a healthy pancreas more closely.
- If needed patient can get a large dose. Just by pressing a switch.
- One needle (to introduce a pump site) every 3–4 days, rather than 3–4 needles a day!

Other ways to take insulin

Beside getting insulin via a syringe there are other devices to get insulin.

Insulin pens

An insulin pen consists of a pen like device filled with insulin that allows you to dial the dose shown in a window and make the injection by pushing in a plunger. Pens come in two different styles:

1) <u>One-time pen.</u> The pen already contains the insulin and is discarded when you use up the insulin.
2) <u>Reusable pen.</u> You put a cartridge of 1.5 or 3 ml of insulin in the pen as needed and can reuse the pen

Many patients find that dialing a dose in an insulin pen is much simpler than taking insulin from a syringe and needle. There are pens containing mixtures if you need mixed type of insulin. Then you don't have to mix two types of insulin.
 Pens are probably the best option for children with T1DM because they're so easy to use and accurate.

A number of different companies make pens. Insulin pens require needles, and you must match the pen with the proper needle in order for the pen to work properly.

The technique for injecting insulin with a pen is the same as injecting with a syringe and needle. The age of your child when you turn injections over to him depends on your assessment of his ability to select the proper dose.

Jet injectors
Jet injectors use a puff of air under pressure to release a jet stream of insulin that's forced through the skin by the pressure of the air. There's no needle involved. You simply draw up the amount of insulin needed, and you can use the device again and again.

Although jet injection devices avoid the use of a needle, they still cause some bruising. For many patients, they're a satisfactory substitute for a syringe and needle. Jet injectors may be used on children, and parents must decide when the child is mature enough to take on the responsibility of administering his own insulin using

the device.
There are several jet injectors available in market to choose from.

Complications of type 1 diabetes?

Type 1 diabetes has short-term complications and long term complications. Short-term complications include hypoglycemia and Diabetic ketoacidosis. In long term complication kidney, heart, vision and nervous system gets affected.

Diabetic ketoacidosis or DKA?

DKA (Diabetic Ketoacidosis) is a dangerous short term complication of Type 1 diabetes. In type 1 diabetes pancreas can't produce insulin. Without insulin, glucose can't enter & work in the cell. This extra Glucose accumulates in blood, causing hyperglycemia.

Glucose is the main source of energy of our body. To function, our body needs glucose. When glucose can't get inside our cells our body starts other option to get energy. To meet this energy demand, stored fat of the body starts to breakdown. Breakdown of fat leads to ketone production. With ketone blood becomes acidic and diabetic ketoacidosis occurs.

DKA is a medical emergency and must be treated at a hospital.

What is the cause of DKA?

The cause of DKA includes
Infection (Pneumonia or lung infection or Urine infection).
Missed insulin injection,
Trauma,
Stroke or
Heart failure.

DKA is a medical emergency, treatment can only be given at hospital / clinic. To confirm DKA a home urine test can be done, which will show deep purple color if high level of ketone is present in urine. In DKA blood sugar is high, more than 250mg/dl (13.8 mmol/L).

To prevent DKA you should never miss insulin injection. Monitor signs of DKA, Child should be trained to recognize symptoms of DKA.

How to recognize DKA?

The good side of DKA (Diabetic Keto Acidosis) is it's easy to recognize if you know the symptoms.

Smell of acetone on the breath: This fruity smell is the smell of the ketone, which are the byproducts of fat breakdown. ketone is excreted in the urine but can be exhaled as well. So fruity Smell of acetone is a major sign of diabetic ketoacidosis.

Confusion or coma: During DKA the thickened, syrupy blood, which is very acidic, circulates through the brain, brain cells are exposed to abnormal byproducts and miss other nutrients that have been lost in the urine. This causes confusion and may proceed to coma.

Cold skin and body temperature: Unless the cause is an infection, the skin is cold as the body's metabolism declines because cells don't get glucose for energy.

Rapid, shallow breathing followed by deep, labored breathing, called Kussmaul breathing after the German doctor who first described it. This unusual breathing pattern is an attempt to blow off some of the acid through the lungs.

Other symptoms are
Increased thirst.
Abdominal pain, Nausea & vomiting.

Ketones: Testing at home

Checking Ketone in urine is confirmatory test of Diabetic Keto Acidosis (DKA) Ketone presence is measured easily by putting a ketone strip into a tube containing urine.

If your or your child's blood glucose is above 250 mg/dl (13.8 mmol/L). You must check urine for ketone.

To do the test, collect urine in a plastic cup and place a ketone strip in urine. The strip will change color. Compare the color with color chart and you get the result. There are four possible results, negative, low, medium or high.

High ketone with high blood glucose mean that your child or you may be on the way to develop DKA (Diabetic ketoacidosis). You should contact your doctor or diabetes health team immediately.

Hypoglycemia diagnosis, and treatment?

Hypoglycemia or low blood glucose is another short-term complication of type 1 diabetes. It is a common but dangerous condition. The good thing is hypoglycemia shows certain symptoms. Which makes it easy to recognize by you or your child.

Hypoglycemia symptoms start to show as soon as blood glucose level becomes 75 mg/dl (4.1 mmol/L) or lower. Symptoms includes Anxiety, Irritability, Numbness in the lips, fingers, and toes.

Cause of hypoglycemia?

Most of the time accidentally taking insulin in high dose causes hypoglycemia. Another cause of hypoglycemia is taking the wrong type of insulin. Other causes are missed meal or small amount of food or too much physical exercise/work.

Some drugs may lower blood glucose leading to hypoglycemia. Such drugs are Beta blockers for hypertension, Aspirin for a headache etc.

Mild hypoglycemia is treated with a small potion of food. Give carbohydrate or sugar containing drinks.

Types of Hypoglycemia and treatment?

When the blood glucose level becomes 65mg/dl (3.6 mmol/L) or lower it's called moderate hypoglycemia. Symptoms include Rapid heartbeat. The sensation of hunger. Sweating and Whiteness or pallor of the skin. Moderate hypoglycemia needs 4 to 5 glucose tablets or oral glucose. Recheck blood glucose after 20 minutes. If blood glucose level is still low give more glucose tablet or powder and recheck again.

When blood glucose level is less than 55 mg/dl (3.05 mmol/L) it's called severe hypoglycemia. Symptoms include Confusion and trouble concentrating, Convulsions, Dizziness, Fatigue, Feeling of warmth, headache, Reduced consciousness or coma, and Slurred speech. Severe hypoglycemia is a medical emergency. You must take the patient to hospital as soon as possible. Give glucagon injection if prescribed by your doctor and available.

There are some common things you can do in any type of hypoglycemia or low blood glucose. If the patient is conscious and can take food by mouth. He should be given 3 to 4 glucose tablets or 15 grams of glucose powder with half glass of water or you can give 15ml or three teaspoons of Honey. Recheck blood glucose 20 minutes later. If the blood glucose level is still low, you can give more glucose tablet or honey.

If the patient is unconscious or unable to take food. Consult your doctor or health care provider.

Instead of glucose tablet (if unavailable). You can give sugar containing drinks such as Apple or orange juice.

Sex and diabetes

Sex is an important part of a healthy relationships. Sex can be an energetic exercise, which means there is a chance of having a hypo either during or after sex. Make sure you have fast-acting glucose nearby. You may also want to tell your partner what to expect if you have a hypo. This could be the time to tell your partner a bit more about diabetes as well.

In the long term, if diabetes is uncontrolled for long time problems while having sex are common complication.

Sexual complications due to T1DM

Uncontrolled T1DM for long time may cause some sexual complications.

Erectile dysfunction (ED) or impotence is the inability to achieve or maintain an erection for sexual intercourse. It is one of the most common sexual problems experienced by men even without diabetes. The main causes are tiredness, stress, emotion, alcohol, smoking, recreational drugs, diabetes, certain medication, surgery and other illnesses.

There is a wide range of treatments for ED including sex therapy, medication (oral, injection and urethral suppository) and vacuum therapy. Less commonly, surgery may be required.

When starting treatment for erection problems it is vital that your diabetes and any other linked conditions such as heart disease are well controlled. Having diabetes does not mean you will go on to develop ED, but it is important to be aware of it in case you experience problems.

Female sexual dysfunction (fSD)
FSD can be caused by physical, emotional and lifestyle factors, medication and diabetes-related complications. Women experiencing FSD may have problems with desire, arousal, pain during intercourse and difficulty achieving orgasm.

Currently there is no medical treatment for FSD, but research is ongoing. Treatments in the form of therapy and aids for lubrication and clitoral stimulation helps.

What is Hypoglycemic unawareness?
Some people with diabetes have no symptoms of hypoglycaemia. They may go severely low or even lose consciousness without even knowing their blood glucose level was dropping. This is known as 'hypoglycemic unawareness'. Hypoglycemic unawareness is a dangerous condition. It occurs in about 25 percent of patients with T1DM. It is dangerous because it causes recurrent sever hypoglycemia. Also it can lead to unconsciousness without any warning symptom.

It occurs more often when one of these risk factors is present:
Many years of diabetes.
Very tight control of the blood glucose.
Frequent and repeated hypoglycemia.

Hypo symptoms can change over time, which may make low blood glucose level harder for you to recognize. No matter the symptoms, always manage low or dropping blood glucose level, even if you feel fine. If you find it hard to recognize hypos, you may need to check your blood glucose level more often – including overnight – and make sure your friends and family know they need to watch for any changes. Make sure your family and friends know what to do when they think you are getting Hypo or become drowsy, disoriented or unconscious. If your normal hypo symptoms disappear or begin to change dramatically, arrange an appointment with your specialist or diabetes educator to discuss what's going on.

Hypoglycemic unawareness is more common during pregnancy, especially in the first trimester. Hypo unawareness can often be overcome by carefully and diligently adjusting insulin and monitoring blood glucose level for a few weeks to avoid further hypoglycaemia during that time.

person with diabetes who suffers frequent severe hypoglycemia can't function normally and is a danger to himself and other. In order to deal with these frequent and severe hypoglycemic reactions, it may be necessary for you to allow the blood glucose to be higher than levels that prevent long-term complications, for example more than 150 mg/dl.

Glucagon injection for hypoglycemia?

Glucagon is a hormone, and it's given in severe hypoglycemia to protect the body.

Glucagon comes in a package containing powder glucagon and water for injection in 2 vials. A syringe with needle is also available. Check the expiration date of glucagon injection.

First, take water from a vial with syringe. Inject the water in the powder containing bottle. Shake to mix powder glucagon with water. Take mixed drug using the syringe and inject into muscle. In hip or upper arm.

Patient and family members should learn the symptoms of hypoglycemia. And how to give glucagon injection.

You need to have glucagon injection, glucose monitoring device and sugar tablet with you at all times.

What happens in hyperglycemia?

Hyperglycemia means height level of glucose in the blood. It happens when we miss an insulin injection. Eating plenty sugar containing food or drinks. Stress or any infection also increases blood glucose.

Excessive blood glucose damage organs of the body such as heart, blood vessels, eyes, nerves etc. High blood glucose affects the body slowly; it causes;

Eye disease -cataract and retinopathy.

Kidney disease - damage the kidneys.

Nervous system damage.

Heart disease.

Diabetic neuropathy

All patients should be screened by doctor for diabetic peripheral neuropathy (DPN) once every year. Symptoms of diabetic nephropathy would be numbness, tingling or burning sensation of hands & foot.

To prevent diabetic neuropathy strictly keeping blood glucose at ideal level is the only option.

Diabetic Eye Disease & Retinopathy

The main eye complications of T1DM are cataracts and retinopathy. Cataracts are opaque areas of the lens of our eyes. Cataracts occur in no more than 1 percent of children with T1DM. In both children and adults, if the cataract is blocking vision, it is removed by surgery and a new lens is implanted, restoring vision.

Retinopathy is considerably more common than cataracts, varying from 15 percent to 50 percent occurrence in patients with T1DM in different studies. It's considerably less common today than it was before the era of intensive diabetic treatment.

This is one of the major long term complication of type 1 diabetes. Retinopathy is classified into two major forms depending on the potential to cause vision loss:

Background retinopathy and Proliferative retinopathy. In both forms, the damage takes place on the retina.

Because diabetic eye disease takes years to develop, the current recommendation is to have your or your child's eyes examined by an ophthalmologist or optometrist when T1DM is first detected. To prevent diabetic retinopathy or eye disease, you must control blood glucose level. Optimize glucose control will reduce the risk or slow the progression of retinopathy.

Diabetic Nephropathy

Uncontrolled blood glucose for a long time or in case of patients with long standing Diabetes a specific kidney disease occurs. It is called diabetic Nephropathy. In Diabetic nephropathy, your kidneys slowly become nonfunctional.

How Diabetic Nephropathy develops?

Kidney disease due to diabetes is known as diabetic nephropathy, and it develops in less than half of the people at risk to get it. There are some factors contribute to kidney disease. Some of these factors you can't change and some of which you can. Following are the factors of diabetic nephropathy;

Abnormal high fats such as cholesterol in blood promote thickening of the kidneys leading to nephropathy. You can reduce this contributing factor by controlling your fat levels present in blood.

Certain ethnic groups, especially African Americans, Native Americans, and Mexican Americans, tend to have nephropathy more often. It's not modifiable.

Elevated blood pressure damages the kidneys of a person with diabetes. Blood pressure should be measured at each doctor's visit and compared with the appropriate chart for age, height, and weight. To prevent diabetic nephropathy, you have to keep your blood pressure controlled level along with your blood sugar.

Preventing Diabetic Nephropathy

The best treatment for kidney disease is preventative. If you can't prevent it with the following measures, you can at least slow it down.

Control your child's or your blood glucose - If you keep your child's blood glucose close to normal, he won't develop diabetic neuropathy. Keep your child's or your blood pressure below the recommended level for age and height.

microalbuminuria is a condition in which minute amount of albumin loss via urine occurs. If you have microalbuminuria, your doctor may prescribe a class of drugs called angiotensin converting enzyme inhibitors. These drugs reverse microalbuminuria while lowering blood pressure.

Control the blood fats by lowering total and bad cholesterol and triglycerides and increasing good cholesterol HDL. Your doctor may prescribe a group of drugs called statins if needed.

People with diabetes tend to have urinary tract infections that can further damage the kidneys, so you or your child needs to drink plenty of fluids. You can acidify the urine with cranberry juice. The bacteria causing urine infection don't like an acidic urine and you can avoid infections.

Nerve damage due to T1DM may cause damage to the nerve for bladder, resulting in a neurogenic bladder with poor emptying of urine and a tendency to develop more urine infection. To prevent Nerve damage good control of your blood glucose is necessary.

In short "To prevent diabetic kidney disease, you must control your blood glucose. Optimize glucose control will reduce the risk or slow the progression of diabetic kidney disease.
You (your child) have to control blood pressure. Keep the blood pressure close to a normal range such as 120 / 80 mmHg. Control fat in the blood. Keep fat level (LDL or HDL) within normal range. Treat urinary infection if you or your child have a urinary infection."

Screening for Diabetic Nephropathy?

Developing diabetic nephropathy takes 10 to 15 years. Alarming thing is, it is a silent development during which there are no clinical signs that the kidneys are failing. But after 15 years of poor control, there are measurable signs of kidney failure as waste products accumulate in the blood, especially blood urea nitrogen and creatinine. This is the stage where significant reduction in kidney filtration but not complete cessation occurs.

By 20 years of poor control, the patient may begin dialysis or needs a kidney transplant in order to survive. So at least every year you should get your urine checked for urinary albumin and estimated glomerular filtration rate (eGFR).

Diet for Diabetic Nephropathy patients.

For people with diabetic kidney disease, reducing the amount of protein in diet is essential.

Skin diseases in T1DM

Many skin conditions are unique to diabetes because of the treatment and complications of the disease. The most common and important skin complications are:

Bruises occur because insulin needles cut blood vessels.

Vitiligo (loss of skin pigmentation) is part of the autoimmune aspect of type 1 diabetes and can't be prevented.

Necrobiosis lipoidica, which also affects people without diabetes, creates patches of reddish-brown skin on the shins or ankles, and the skin becomes thin and ulcerated. Females tend to have this condition more often than males. Steroid injections are used to treat this condition, and the areas eventually become depressed and brown.

Xanthelasma, which are small, yellow, flat areas called plaques on the eyelids, occur in type 1 diabetes even when cholesterol isn't elevated. Treatment may not be necessary.

Alopecia, or loss of hair, occurs in people with type 1 diabetes, but the cause is unknown.

Insulin hypertrophy is the accumulation of fatty tissue where insulin is injected. This condition is prevented by changing the injection site regularly.

Insulin lipoatrophy is the loss of fat where the insulin is injected. Although the cause is unknown, this condition is rarely seen now that human insulin has replaced beef and pork insulin in diabetes treatment.

Diabetic thick skin is thicker than normal skin, occurs in people who have had diabetes for more than ten years.

Are you more prone to illness when You have Diabetes?

A common misconception is that people with T1DM are more prone to illness. This is not true.

If you compare frequency of illness in the population with T1DM with that of people who don't have diabetes, there's no difference between them. People with T1DM get viral illnesses no more often than those without T1DM. This myth about being prone to illness is a popular one that originated when T1DM was so hard to treat, before 1921.

Though T1DM patients are not prone to illness, but the complications of any illness is more in T1DM. So they need to take a flu shot every year to prevent the severe illness that may be associated with that disease. Elderly people with T1DM especially should get shots for pneumonia and shingles. But during flu or other illness you have to adjust insulin intake, modify diet, and take medicine carefully.

Steps for Reducing complications of diabetes.

Manage diabetes. Keep your blood glucose, blood pressure and cholesterol at target levels.

Regularly test your blood glucose level. For type 1 diabetes it's at least 3 times daily before meals.

See your doctor for all your recommended screening tests.

Take your prescribed medicine regularly.

Quit smoking.

Exercise at least 30 min every alternate day.

Follow a diet plan. Consult a dietitian for specific diet plan for you.

Limit alcohol intake.

Maintain ideal weight.

What you need learn to help your child with T1DM?

The major skills that you must acquire to help your child and skills that your child must learn as he grows includes the following:
Understanding the diabetes disease process and the options for treatment including ways of administering insulin, diet, exercise, and so forth.

You must learn adjusting to the psychosocial demands of T1DM.

Learn to monitoring blood glucose and urine ketones and using the results to improve glucose control.

Learn managing nutrition.

Learn incorporating physical activity in the child's lifestyle.

Learn using insulin properly.

Learn preventing, detecting, and treating acute complications (DKA, Hypo etc.)

Learn preventing, detecting, and treating chronic complications (retinopathy, neuropathy etc.)

Learn setting goals to promote health, and problem solving for daily living.

Learn preconception care and management during pregnancy.

Learn care and management for the elderly.

How to deal with a child with type 1 diabetes?

Type 1 diabetes, mainly occurs in children. It's difficult to explain the condition to your child. You have to teach him to live with the disease and have a positive attitude.

Let the child take control of his diabetes, let him or her decided what should be eaten, how much play or exercise is good.

Appreciate achievements such as normal blood sugar, healthy eating.

Teach him to recognize the symptoms of complication.

You and your child must understand that it is not possible to control every high blood glucose. The true goal of type 1 diabetes is to keep overall control of blood glucose level.

Explain to your child that many successful people have diabetes. Diabetes does not have any effect on IQ or good looks. By giving your child a positive attitude you can lead him to a successful life.

Caring for children with Type 1 Diabetes of specific ages

Children with Type 1 diabetes have different reaction to diabetes at different age. Young children passively but not happily accept the insulin shots, whereas young adults want to take charge of their condition.

Infants up to 18 months

Most of the time diagnosis of Type 1 diabetes is missed in infants. Infants can't tell about their problems. You have to look for the symptoms like frequent diaper change due to increased urination. Persistent vomiting is also a sign of type 1 diabetes. Consult your doctor for a screening test of type 1 diabetes.

The infant up to 18 months of age with T1DM is completely under the care of his parent (usually the mother). He'll resist his shots and his glucose tests but you must clearly understand that they're essential. This is something you have to insist upon even though the child can't understand the reason.

It's best for the baby's neurological system to allow his blood glucose to be a little higher than normal. A blood glucose between 150 and 200 mg/dl (8.3 to 11.1 mmol/L) is a good target upto 2 years of age.

Toddlers between 18 months and 3 years

The toddler who is 18 months to 3 years old is at the stage of beginning to test his parents, establishing himself as a separate human being. He's starting to learn to control his environment (by toilet training, for example). With diabetes, he may refuse shots, refuse to eat enough and at the right time, and generally make it difficult for you to manage the disease. You have to set limits and be firm, know when to insist when the item is essential (like taking insulin) and when to give in so that the child can have some victories as well (like allowing the child a piece of birthday cake).

Use of very short-acting insulin is helpful in toddlers because the child's eating habits tend to be irregular and you can give the insulin just as the child begins to eat.

Children between 3 and 6 years

The child between ages 3 and 6 is still home and tests your limitations even more than a toddler. But he can tell you when he has symptoms of hypoglycemia. At this age, the child is wondering what he did to deserve diabetes when all his friends don't have it. Get the child involved with food preparation so that he feels he plays a part in his care. As your child gets closer to 6 years old, think about enrolling him in a diabetes camp or a children's diabetes group. There he'll be surrounded by kids like him and will realize that everyone has similar concerns and limitations.

Don't try to teach your young child about the complications of diabetes yet. He doesn't possess the skills or knowledge to manage his disease and will simply be frightened.

Children between 6 and 12 years

As the child begins school between 6 and 12 years of age, he wants to know more. This is the time for you and the child to go to a diabetes education program and to sit down together with a dietitian to work out the best diet to promote continued growth and good diabetic control. It's also the time to hand over some of the control (don't give up control of the insulin just yet), especially because you're not at school to monitor the child all the time. Establish that the school has food that's healthy for your child and also has a program where knowledgeable people are available to help him in the event of hypoglycemia.

Teens between 13 and 15 years
When the child reaches age 13 to 15 and officially becomes a teenager, he's extremely curious and wants to know about everything, including his diabetes. Another trip together to a diabetes education program and the dietitian is essential. At this age, involving both parents in diabetes education and treatment is even better than just 1 parent.

This and the following stage may be a very difficult time in terms of trying to keep good glucose control because of the production of large amounts of growth hormone, which tends to raise blood glucose. Don't expect perfect blood glucose level.

Teens between 15 and 19
The stage of puberty, from age 15 to 19, with all the new and powerful hormones (especially the sex hormones) may prove to be the most difficult time of all to manage T1DM. All the problems of attraction to and being attractive for a significant other seem to get in the way.

Tips for Parents of T1DM.
Learn as much as you can on Diabetes. Use internet, medical handout and books on T1DM.
Talk with your child. Give him/her courage. Teach him / her self-care for diabetes.

Make sure your child wears a medical identification product such as bracelet or pendant.

Communicate with school health team. Talk to school nurse.

Give school an emergency contact address and Cell phone number.

Provide all necessary items needed to maintain your child's health plan.

Ideal body weight for type 1 diabetes?

Managing and keeping ideal weight is essential for any diabetic patient. Balanced weight lowers the chance of heart and kidney disease.

To understand ideal body weight, we have to know Body Mass Index or BMI. It's calculated by dividing your weight in Kilograms by your height in meter squared. A BMI below 18.5 is underweight. A BMI from 18.5 to 24.99 is the ideal weight. BMI 30 or more is obese.

Try to keep your BMI in the normal range. If your BMI is high, try to lose 5 -10% of your body weight. Be sure to consult with your doctor and approach the weight loss gradually. Remember, you should not start any weight loss program or diet without consulting your doctor.

Type 1 diabetic patients tend to be underweight and malnourished. The underweight body makes it difficult to stay healthy. Consult your dietitian for advice on how to gain weight. Some weight gain tips are, eat small but frequent meals. Add more fat (margarine, cheese, butter, oil, etc.) to your diet. Eat dried fruit and nuts.

Do you have to eat special foods in Type 1 Diabetes?

With T1DM, there's no advantage of eating special diabetic foods. It's difficult enough to deal with all the requirements for good diabetes care. Restriction of Food will be too much. Food is one of life's great pleasures, and your child can have excellent glucose control with regular food so long as you know how much carbohydrate is in it.

Then you can adjust the dose of insulin to cover the extra carb. Show your child that he can eat delicious meals and still follow his diet plan. Prepare meals that the whole family can eat. There's no reason that everyone in the family shouldn't eat the same meals as your child with T1DM.

Now on off the shelf products, people assume that if the label says 'diabetic' that the contents may be beneficial for diabetics. But it's not true all the time. Since 'diabetic' foods tend to cost more than conventional counterparts or sugar-free and reduced sugar versions, this is in effect conning people with diabetes.

For example, Diabetic Chocolate – "is sweetened with alcohol sugars, which can cause fluid to build up in your bowels, which can then cause diarrhoea"

So go for normal products and chocolate but in moderate quantity.

Food for type 1 diabetes?

Food is a major component in the treatment of type 1 diabetes. It is important to consult with a dietitian for a personalized diet plan.

Bread, rice, potatoes, pasta & other starchy foods are the source of carbohydrate. Carbohydrate is broken down to simple sugar in our body. It gives us all the energy we need. But carbohydrate is also the main source of glucose in the blood. We should watch how much carbohydrate we take with each meal. 40 to 60 percent of calories of our diet should come from carbohydrate.

Meat, fish, eggs, beans are sources of protein. Protein is needed for repair and growth of our body. Proteins do not have a direct effect on blood glucose. It is the main component of hormones, enzymes and antibodies. 10 to 20 percent of calories of our diet should come from protein. As part of a mixed meal, protein will slow the absorption of carbohydrate. Which is good for you.

Milk & dairy foods have essential vitamins and minerals. These products also have an effect on blood glucose.

Fruit & vegetables They contain essential vitamins. For a healthy diet fruit and vegetables are essential.

What is Carbohydrate counting

Carbohydrate counting is a calculation of total carbohydrate in your or your child's meal. Carbohydrate counting is used to determine how much insulin is needed to balance your meal. The key to this system is knowing the carbohydrate in your food. A dietitian is needed initially. The dietitian will know your food preferences and tell you how many grams of carbohydrate are in them.

For carbohydrate counting, you also need to know how many grams of carbohydrate are controlled by each unit of insulin you or your child takes. This is determined by checking blood glucose one hour after eating a known amount of carbohydrate. It varies person to person. For example, one person may need 1 unit of rapid-acting insulin to control 20 grams of carbohydrate, whereas another person may need 2 unit.

Advantage of carbohydrate counting is that your child can eat a variety of foods as long as you know the carbohydrate count of what he's eating. Children who are allowed this process are much happier with their food, and their hemoglobin A1cs are significantly lower.

INTERESTING FACT

In general, 1 unit of rapid-acting insulin is needed to control 15 grams of carbohydrate.

What is Glycemic Index or GI index?

It's a way to rank foods on how fast they can rise your blood sugar. The top of GI Index is 100 which is pure glucose. Actual GI Index for every food makes it difficult to apply in real life. So foods are labeled as low GI food (Index less than 55) or high GI food (Index more then 70).

High GI food (Index more then 70) Bad choice for T1DM because; It Make blood sugars rise & fall rapidly. But it is a good choice when hypoglycaemia occur.
Long grain rice, although a complex carbohydrate actually has a high GI. On the other hand, basmati rice has a much lower GI.

Low GI foods (Index less than 55) is good choice for T1DM because it makes blood sugar levels rise slowly and remain in our system for a long period of time. It is a good choice to have as main meal or before exercise.
Low GI foods with large particles that our bodies take a long time to digest and hence release their energy slowly. Example of this type of food are; lentils, soy beans, cherries, yoghurt, oats, pasta, grainy breads etc.

How to switch to a low GI Diet: If you want to get into the GI diet, it's really about choices like knowing that blood sugars will fluctuate less by having multigrain instead of white bread, having pasta instead of rice, and having oat based cereals.

The main things to concentrate on if you'd like to go low GI are:
Use breakfast cereals based on oats, barley and bran;
Use 'grainy' breads made with whole seeds;
Make use of pasta and traditional (not easy to cook) and basmati rice in your meals;
Be aware that potatoes have a higher GI and if you include a low GI vegetable like peas or beans with your potatoes this will lower the GI

of your entire meal. Or you could substitute sweet potato which has a much lower GI.

Enjoy all types of fruit and vegetables;

Include plenty of salads (especially bean-based ones) with vinaigrette dressing.

All dairy products have a low GI. A glass of milk before bed, will provide a slow release of energy and prevent overnight hypoglycemia.

Goals of Nutrition Therapy for Adults with Diabetes

Goal one- Get a healthy and nutritious meal. Your food choice will help you achieve your desired blood glucose level, ideal body weight, target blood pressure. Your food choice will help you to prevent complications of diabetes.

Goal two – maintain the pleasure of eating. With type 1 diabetes there is no restriction on what you eat, it's how much you eat is important. There is no restriction on what you eat. A good nutrition therapy will restore the pleasure of eating.

Goal three – a nutrition therapy will provide the individual with diabetes practical tools for day-to-day meal planning.

Tips on food.

Food is an essential part of type 1 diabetes treatment. It's best to consult with a dietitian to get your personalized diet plan. There are some common tips to help you with your diet.

Eat more whole grains, fruits, & veggies.

Limit or avoid foods that are high in fat, sugar, and white flour.

Always use low-fat milk, cheese, yogurt and dairy products.

Use pulses such as peas, beans or lentils to replace or reduce meat.

Cut and remove visible fat from meat, from poultry product remove skin.

When cooking, try to drain excess fat from meat before adding spices.

Try to grill or baking instead frying.

Learn low-fat cooking methods.

Eat carbohydrate that is slow to absorb with low glycemic Index.

Eat pasta, basmati or easy cook rice, grainy bread such as granary, pumpernickel, rye, new potatoes, sweet potato, yam porridge, oats and natural muesli. These foods have low glycemic index so blood glucose will be low.

For fat Choose unsaturated fats or oils, such as olive, rapeseed and sunflower oil. These fat will help you to lose weight. You can reach your target cholesterol level with low fat diet.

Use less butter, margarine and cheese.

Eat fish at least once every week.

Eat 1 potion of fruit such as 1 apple or banana or any other fruit you like every day.

Avoid sugary drinks or smoothies.

Do not take more than 6g of salt per day. Less salt reduces blood pressure and heart disease.

Do not take alcohol more than 3 units per day. Half a pint of lager, ale, bitter or cider has 1-1½ units. Do not take alcohol on an empty stomach.

Required carbohydrate for a child.

Child male or female age 5 to 10 years needs 200 grams to 270 grams' carbohydrate every day.

Male child age 11 to 15 needs 270 grams to 400 grams of carbohydrate daily. And a female child of 11 to 15 years needs 275 to 300 grams of carbohydrate daily.

A female child of 16 to 18 years needs 250 to 300 grams of carbohydrate daily. A male child of 16 to 18 years need 300 to 475 grams of carbohydrate per day.

Tips on carbohydrate.

Eat and teach your child to eat carbohydrate (rice, pasta, etc.) in large chunks. It takes time to breakdown large piece of carbohydrate inside our gut. So glucose is absorbed slowly and blood glucose rises slowly.

Eat carbohydrate with fat to slow down absorption. When we eat carbohydrates with fat, the fat slows down the movement of food through the intestine, so the blood glucose rises more slowly.

Small snacks in between meals can keep your blood glucose at a consistent level which is good for your diabetes.

Whole fruit, like an orange, requires breakdown of cell walls in the intestine, but that breakdown has already occurred in orange juice. So carbohydrate in orange juice is absorbed more rapidly than the carbohydrate in a whole orange. The same is true of finely ground flour, as found in white bread compared with whole-grain bread. So whole fruit instead of juice and whole grain bread is good choice.

Drinking a beverage with a meal makes the food pass more rapidly into the intestine where it's absorbed, so blood glucose rises more rapidly. Avoid beverage with main meals. When you need a rapid rise of blood glucose (in case of hypoglycemia) drink fruit juice or any beverage with food.

Light exercise like walking speeds up the absorption of glucose, whereas heavy exercise like running slows it down.

Very cold or hot food slows down the emptying of the stomach, thus slowing the absorption of glucose.

A high blood glucose slows the emptying of the stomach, whereas a low blood glucose speeds it up.

Tips on Protein.

A gram of protein contains 4 kilocalories. Protein is the second major source of calories of our diet, it is found in the muscles of animals (beef, poultry, and fish), cheese, eggs, and milk. It's usually accompanied by more or less fat, depending upon the source.

Protein in a meal doesn't contribute to blood glucose immediately. It takes several hours for protein to be converted into sugar in the body unless the blood glucose is low, in which case the conversion happens much more rapidly.

You should be selecting low-fat sources of protein for your child, developing his palate so that he enjoys food without fat. Following are some fast facts about sources of protein:

The protein sources with the least amount of fat, only 1 gram per ounce of protein are very lean meat or fish and fat-free cheese. Shellfish like lobster and shrimp are also included in this category.

Lean protein with 3 grams of fat per ounce includes lean beef and pork, dark meat chicken, oily fish like salmon, and some cheese. These sources of protein are still a good choice for your child, especially oily fish because the fat in it is omega-3 fatty acid, which has beneficial effects on the heart. Serve your family a minimum of two meals of oily fish per week so that everyone gets enough omega-3 fatty acid.

The categories of medium-fat proteins with 5 grams of fat per ounce and high-fat proteins with 8 grams of fat per ounce include foods that should be limited in your child's diet because of the very high fat content. Fried foods, processed sandwich meats, regular fat meats, and very fatty meats like bacon and pork are in these category.

Eating a lot of protein in the medium- to high-fat category will cause weight gain, and the fat in these foods is the kind that raises cholesterol and worsens arteriosclerosis means hardening of the arteries. It's bad for you.

Another factor to consider when selecting protein sources is the amount of mercury. In certain fish the mercury content is high. Regularly eating fish with high levels of mercury can lead to mercury poisoning and is especially bad for young children and pregnant and nursing mothers. The fish with the most mercury that you should avoid are shark, swordfish, mackerel, and tilefish.

For several reasons, experts feel strongly about limiting protein in the diet to 20 percent of calories One reason is the fat that's consumed with the protein, although choosing low-fat sources of protein reduces this problem.
Another reason is that although higher levels of protein haven't been shown to hurt normal kidneys, they do seem to worsen the damage in kidneys that are failing. Study showed that a diet very low in protein could postpone the need for dialysis in all patients with chronic kidney disease.

Tips on Fat.

Fat has more than twice as many calories per gram as carbohydrate and protein. But it doesn't have a direct immediate effect on the blood glucose level. Consumed to excess, it causes weight gain, and increased weight results in resistance to insulin. In fact, as I mention earlier, fat in a meal may lower blood glucose by slowing the absorption of the glucose.

It's different in case of children. Children need a lot of fat in their diet up until the age of 5. Breast milk is 50 percent fat, for example. After the age of 5, children should begin eating a diet of less fat, with the emphasis on types of fat that decrease the development of arteriosclerosis rather than increase it. The fats to avoid are saturated fats and trans fats.

When a child is over age 5, the recommended daily intake of fat is 30 percent of kilocalories and no more than 300 mg of cholesterol in the diet. That much cholesterol is found in an egg yolk. An ounce of hard cheese like cheddar has 28 mg of cholesterol, and a glass of whole milk has 35 mg of cholesterol. Switch your child to skim milk and you drop to just 5 mg of cholesterol.

In addition to cholesterol, fat comes as several forms of triglyceride.

Saturated fat raises a person's cholesterol level and worsens arteriosclerosis. It's the main fat in meat, but it's also present in certain vegetable oils, especially coconut oil, palm oil, and palm kernel oil.

If your child must have that occasional steak, encourage him to cut off all visible fat.

Trans fatty acid, though present in nature, is mostly added to foods by food manufacturers looking to replace butter. The trouble is that trans fatty acids not only raise LDL (bad) cholesterol, but they lower HDL (good) cholesterol at the same time, so they are even worse than butter!

Unsaturated fat is a much better choice than saturated fat and trans fatty acids because it doesn't raise bad cholesterol. You can choose monounsaturated fat, which is in avocado, olive oil, canola oil, and nuts like almonds and peanuts. Or polyunsaturated fat, which is in soft fats and oils such as corn oil, mayonnaise, and margarine. Keep in mind polyunsaturated fat lowers good cholesterol. So the best choice is monounsaturated fat.

Fat should make up 30 percent of your child's daily caloric intake, and most of that 30 percent should be from the unsaturated fat group.

Oatmeal lowers the bad cholesterol but also contains soluble fiber, so it slows the absorption of glucose.

Apples and pears make good snacks because they also provide soluble fiber.

A handful of walnuts or almonds is a great snack that reduces bad cholesterol. But don't overdo the nuts — the "good" fat in them is still fat and has 9 kilocalories per gram.

Delicious salmon provides the omega-3 fatty acids described in the previous section on protein to lower triglycerides. Walnuts, canola oil, and soybean oil have omega-3s that do the same.

Soy protein, once thought to have cholesterol-lowering power, has now been shown to have little effect on the cholesterol.

Tips on Vitamins.

Vitamins and minerals are food substances that the body needs in minute quantities. Luckily, a balanced diet usually provides all these in sufficient amounts

Vitamin A Needed for healthy skin and bones, source of vitamin A are Milk and green vegetables.

Vitamin B1 (thiamin) Converts carbohydrates into energy, found in Meat and wholegrain cereals.

Vitamin B2 (riboflavin) Needed to use food properly, found in Milk, cheese, fish, and green vegetables.

Vitamin B6 (pyridoxine) Needed for growth found in Liver, yeast, potatoes, bananas, and chicken breasts

Vitamin B12 Keeps the red blood cells and the nervous system healthy, found in animal foods, such as meat, dairy products and eggs.

Folic acid Keeps the red blood cells and the nervous system healthy available in Green vegetables.

Niacin Helps release energy available in Lean meat, fish, nuts, and legumes.

Vitamin C Helps maintain supportive tissues found in Fruits and potatoes.

Vitamin D Helps with absorption of calcium found Dairy products.

Vitamin E Helps maintain cells balanced available in Vegetable oils and whole-grain cereals.

Vitamin K Needed for proper clotting of the blood get it from Leafy vegetables

A note to keep in mind that Kids don't need vitamin pills (nor do most adults) if they eat a healthy diet. Only in cases in which the body rapidly uses food and vitamins, as in pregnancy or acute illness there is a possibility that the person doesn't get enough of these vitamins. Then a supplemental vitamin pills a good choice. Otherwise, it's just a waste of money.

Tips on Minerals.

Minerals provide basic structure in your child's body, and he may need extra amounts of them to ensure that he gets enough. This is true for any child, not just one with T1DM. Here are a few important minerals for both children and adults:

Calcium, phosphorus, and magnesium: These minerals build bones and teeth. Fortunately, children get enough of them from milk and other dairy products. Adults, especially women, usually need to supplement their calcium intake by taking calcium tablets.

Iron: This mineral is a major component of hemoglobin in red blood cells. Spinach is considered a good source of iron, as are other leafy green vegetables. Other good sources are meat, beans, and seafood. As your daughter with T1DM begins to menstruate, she loses iron each time she bleeds. It's important to make sure she gets foods with extra iron.

Sodium: This mineral helps to regulate body water. It seems like everything has salt in it naturally, and it's pretty difficult to avoid consuming too much, especially if you ever take your child to a fast-food place. Teach your child to enjoy the taste of food without added salt. His blood pressure will benefit. Don't put salt on the table at mealtimes, and don't use too much of it in cooking.

Chromium: This mineral, which is found in whole grains, bran cereals, and potatoes, is often claimed to be missing in people with diabetes. There is a myth you will know and on the internet that chromium is used to treat and cure diabetes.
This claim is a myth Scientific literature still hasn't proven this point. Studies done with chromium doesn't look promising.

Iodine: This mineral is a critical part of the thyroid hormones. If your child eats any kind of bread, he gets enough iodine because the bread usually is fortified with iodized salt.

Various other minerals, like chlorine, cobalt, tin, and zinc: These minerals are found in many foods. There is very little likelihood that a child will be deficient in any of them, which generally are required in very small amounts.

Understanding Diet at Every Age

Children with T1DM should follow the nutritional guidelines from a professional dietitian but as with all children, diet challenges can arise. Here are some issues that you may face as your child grows.

The newborn: Hopefully, the newborn is breast-feeding, but if breastfeeding isn't possible, formula may be used for a baby with T1DM. It's unusual for a newborn to develop T1DM, but should it occur, the high fat content of breast milk (50 percent fat) will result in very slow absorption of the sugar in milk. Short-acting insulin should be given before each breast or formula feeding. Very small amounts of insulin are required, sometimes measured in half units.

The toddler: A child at this age may be a picky eater, but he'll probably eat enough to grow normally. It may be necessary to determine the dose and give insulin after the child has eaten so that you know how many grams of carbohydrate have been consumed. Toddlers often don't feel hungry early in the morning, so breakfast may be missed. If glucose is needed for low blood glucose, giving it in a gel form may be better than a tablet because the gel doesn't have to be chewed.

Preschooler: A child at this age is beginning a growth spurt that will last the next 15 years. A preschooler's activity level and food intake is very erratic, so it's hard to predict the correct insulin dosage.

Therefore, attempting to control the blood glucose in a child this age is difficult.

Preschoolers obtain a large amount of their energy from fat rather than carbohydrates. They don't do well on high-fiber foods, which upset their stomachs. They may use food as a way of gaining some control, which makes feeding them even more difficult. Try to give your preschooler with T1DM a choice in what he eats, and praise him for good eating behavior. Never force-feed your child if you think he isn't getting enough calories. It's usually best to give a preschooler insulin after eating because you know how much carbohydrate he has eaten.

Primary school: For children who are at the age of entering school, diet challenges shift from the home environment to the school because the children spend so much time at school and eat at least one meal there. It's necessary to work with the school dietitian to set up a good meal program. One thing that may make control easier is the regimentation of the school environment and the tendency to serve the same thing on a regular basis.

Someone at the school has to be able to determine how much insulin should be given and give it. It's better to err on the side of too little than too much insulin. At this age, your child is increasingly active, and this has to be taken into account when determining the insulin dose. It may be easier to control his diabetes if the meals are smaller and the snacks more numerous, thus reducing the amount of insulin needed at any one time.

Puberty from 13 to 19 years of age: Children at this age are much more capable of understanding the importance of good control of the blood glucose and, hopefully, will adopt the eating habits that make control easier. At this age, your child is under the influence of many hormones that tend to raise the blood glucose, especially growth hormone, so insulin needs may be higher. At the same time, he's doing his best not to stick out, so if the group goes for candy, he will too. Lapses like this will certainly make glucose control more difficult.

Children with T1DM generally know what they need to eat to grow normally and stop eating when they're no longer hungry. You can always check that this is the case for your child by comparing him with the standard height and weight tables for his age.

Using sugar substitutes

Before the isolation of insulin in 1921, sugar was thought to be extremely dangerous for the person with T1DM. With nothing available to lower the blood sugar, consuming sugar actually was pretty dangerous. By completely cutting sugar from the diet of these patients was the only treatment option.

Old habits take a long time to die, and there are still plenty of people, even doctors, who think that people with diabetes must avoid sugar at all costs. Most physicians no longer believe this and permit some sugar in the diet of patients with T1DM, but the wish to avoid sugar has created an industry of products with fewer or no calories yet great sweetening power.

You can use sweeteners for your child with T1DM by substituting one for sugar in a recipe, but you need to know their sweetening power to use them correctly.

Sugar-free food can still have plenty of fat and protein calories. Because total calories are what counts in the diet, there's no great advantage to eating sugar free products when the result may be that your child's getting as many or more total calories.

Calorie-containing sweeteners

This group consists of a sugar similar to glucose and the so-called sugar alcohols. Fructose has the same number of kilocalories per gram as glucose, but the sugar alcohols have half as many. Food manufacturers like to use the sugar alcohols in all kinds of products that they call "sugarless," but it's important to remember that the sugar alcohols aren't calorie-free. Here's a rundown of fructose and sugar alcohols:

Fructose is fruit sugar found in fruits and berries. Its great advantage it that it's absorbed much more slowly than glucose although it has about the same sweetening power as table sugar.
Xylitol is a sugar alcohol found in strawberries and raspberries. Xylitol has the sweetening power of sucrose. It's taken up slowly from the intestine, so it causes little change in blood glucose. Xylitol doesn't cause cavities of the teeth as often as the other sweeteners containing calories, so it's commonly used in chewing gum, hard candy, and some drugs.

Sorbitol and mannitol are sugar alcohols occurring in plants. Sorbitol and mannitol are half as sweet as table sugar and have little effect on blood glucose. They change to fructose in the body. When taken as a food, sorbitol doesn't accumulate and damage tissues. Sorbitol is used in candies, chewing gum, jams and jellies, and baked goods. Mannitol is used in chewing gum, candies, jams and jellies, and frostings.

Non-nutritive or artificial sweeteners
These sweeteners contain no calories yet are much sweeter than sucrose by weight. Several of them have been very controversial as far as the possibility that they cause cancer. As a result, the Food and Drug Administration (FDA) has developed the concept of acceptable daily intake, or ADI. This is the maximum daily intake that's safe to consume each day over a lifetime.
The ADIs in the following list are for adults. The ADI for a child is based on the size of a child compared to an average adult. For example, if the average adult is 150 pounds, the ADI for a 75-pound

child is half the adult value.

Aspartame: It's 150 to 200 times sweeter than sucrose. Many people seem to prefer the taste of aspartame. It is used in diet soda and beverages. It has an ADI of 18 to 19 cans of diet soda. It's not useful for cooking.

Acesulfame: This sweetener is 200 times sweeter than sucrose and doesn't leave an aftertaste. It can be used in cooking and is found in numerous foods and beverages as well as a tabletop sweetener. It has an ADI of 30 to 32 cans of diet soda.

Saccharin: This sweetener is 300 to 400 times sweeter than sucrose. It comes in packets. The ADI for saccharin is 9 to 12 packets per day.

Sucralose: This sweetener is obtained from sugar and is 600 times sweeter. It's very stable and can be used in place of sugar in any food. It leaves no unpleasant aftertaste. As its available in diet soda Its ADI is six cans of diet soda.

Physical Activity for type 1 diabetes.

Children with type 1 diabetes must engage in physical activity at least for 60 min every day. He should do Aerobic exercise, muscle strengthening and bone strengthening exercise at least three times every week.

For adults at least 150 min physical activity per week is a must. Adults with type 1 diabetes should engage in physical activity such as aerobic exercise every alternate day. Gradually increase the amount of physical activity that you do each day until you reach 30-60 minutes of continuous activity.

You or your child should get up and walk for a brief time when you are inactive or desk bound for more than 90 min. Time spent in sedentary styles such as TV, computer or mobile games should be broken into small segments of less than 90 min. Teach your child to get up, move or do small physical activity during a commercial break in case of watching TV. During a game on computer or mobile or tab teach him to take small breaks after each level.

School with type 1 diabetes?

Child or adult everyone who has type 1 diabetes must wear Medical Alert ID (as bracelet or pendant.)

Always carry glucose tablet, energy bar, glucometer with lancet & strip, insulin with syringe and glucagon kit. Make two or three small pack which has everything needed. keep the pack all time with you. Stick post it note on your door and mirror to remind you not to forget your diabetic pack.

Know how to contact school health team.

Discard your lancets and syringe in proper container.

Do not miss insulin injection and meals.

At school a Diabetic child should have these things with him all the time.

Diabetes management plans and prescriptions.

Monitoring equipment (e.g. lancets, meter strips, alcohol, ketone strips).

Glucose tablets or other fast-acting forms of carbohydrate to treat hypoglycemia.

Insulin and related supplies (e.g. insulin pump supplies or insulin syringes and/or pen).

Ketone monitoring supplies.

Glucagon kit.

Parents responsibility of school going child with type 1 diabetes?

You should notify school principal and school health team about the condition of your child.

Give your correct and current contact information. Remember to update the information when you change your address or ph1 number.

Participate in meetings of school health team.

Visiting your doctor?

Even if there are no physical complications, you or your child should visit a doctor or diabetes health team every six months'.

If any complication occurs, you must consult your doctor immediately.

Your doctor will check blood pressure on every visit. The target blood pressure is lower than 130/80mmHg.

Doctor will check your foot for damage or ulcers (vascular damage).

If your child is 10 years or older, your doctor will check the eyes for damage caused by Diabetes (Diabetic retinopathy). Every 2 years he will check and take a picture of the retina with a device called funduscope

He will check your urine and run some blood test to see the condition of your kidneys (Diabetic Nephropathy).

He would check your nervous system for numbness in hands and legs (Diabetic Neuropathy).

These are painless physical exams done by your doctor or diabetes health team from time to time. It helps in early diagnosis if you or your child has any complications of diabetes.

Type 1 diabetic patients' checkup every 6 months' even if there are no specific complaints.

Every six months Check:

Blood pressure

Weight

Body mass index

Waist circumference

Foot care

Every year check:

HbA1c

Total cholesterol, LDL cholesterol and triglycerides

Kidney check (urine micro albumin test)

Medication review

Smoking status

Healthy eating plan

Physical activity

Self-care education

At least every two years:

Eye examination (more frequently if evidence of disease)

Please note that these recommendations may be different in your country. It may be different for children or young adults.

Some myths about Diabetes

There is a common myth that diabetic patients can't have sugar or chocolate. This is not true. Diabetes patients can have sugar or chocolate but has to adjust the insulin dose to control the extra sugar. But It's best to avoid sugar and sugar-containing foods as much as possible.

Another myth is diabetic people can't play sports. It's also a misconception. A well-controlled Diabetic can play sports and do physical Exercise. It's even good for him. But he should be careful with low blood glucose (hypoglycemia) and keep glucometer and some glucose tablet and glucagon kit handy.

Smoking and Type 1 Diabetes

Smoking is a major health hazard even without diabetes. With diabetes, smoking creates many complications. You have to quit smoking, there is no other option. You already know what are the bad effects of smoking so I am taking another approach.

Following are the benefits of quitting smoke.

Only 20 minutes after quitting you heart rate and blood pressure improve.

In 8 hours' nicotine is out of your body, oxygen level of your blood improves. With oxygen, you feel stronger and healthy.

In 48 hours of quitting your sense of smell and test improve dramatically.

In a month, you become healthier with reduced chance of heart attack and stroke.
In three months your breathing improves. Chronic cough and cold are reduced just in 3 months after quitting.

In 6 months your skin will improve. You will look younger and feel younger.

Immunization for Type 1 Diabetes patient

Take all routine vaccinations; other vaccinations for T1DM are;

You or your child (if more than 6 months of age) should get Influenza vaccination every year.

You or your child (more than 2 years old) must get Pneumococcal polysaccharide vaccine 23 or PPSV23 vaccine.

Adults 65 or more years of age, should get Pneumococcal conjugate vaccine 13 (PCV13), followed by PPSV23 6–12 months after initial vaccination. If not previously vaccinated.

Get hepatitis B vaccination.

Maintaining a Quality Life with type 1 diabetes.

To have a quality life and maintain it with Type 1 Diabetes you have to control your or your child's blood glucose level, blood pressure and blood cholesterol level. The keys to maintaining a high quality of life with T1DM are;

Regular measuring of blood glucose and knowing how to respond to high and low blood glucose.

Get regular examination (6 months to every year) by your doctor or healthcare professional.

Learn how to count carbohydrate quantity in meals and adjust insulin dose accordingly.

Enjoying good food that's also nutritious.

Exercise regularly to keep your muscles in excellent shape This will help to keep your metabolism functioning well.

Get sufficient sleep at least 8 hours every day.
Avoiding blaming you or your child when things don't go exactly as you planned.

Parents of Type 1 Diabetic child.

As a parent there are few things you can do to improve the life of your child with type 1 diabetes.

Maintain a balance between control and freedom. If you pressurize the child to control every high blood glucose. It will stress him out. He will rebel and stop following advice. So focus on overall correction of blood glucose.

Anger in child with type 1 diabetes is a natural response. He becomes angry with all the limitation due to type 1 diabetes. Talk to your child. Try to find out the specific cause of anger. Sometimes you should give your child some freedom from strict routine lifestyle.

Be aware that neither you nor your child is to blame for the fact that he or you have diabetes. T1DM doesn't result from consuming too much sugar, failing to exercise sufficiently, or any other failure that you may imagine.

Don't overreact to any temporary loss of control or increased glucose level of your child. Try to find the cause. Control of the blood glucose may be lost temporarily when your child gets sick with a virus or other problems. When it happens, move on and try to restore the control as soon as possible. Do not blame the child. A child who's really trying but gets blamed when things go wrong will quickly lose interest in trying.

Recognize that depression can occur in patients with type 1 diabetes. If your child's sleep is disturbed, if he doesn't want to eat, if his usual positive outlook changes to sadness and unhappiness, it may be the time to consult your psychiatrist.

Know when to begin turning over control of the day-to-day management of diabetes to the child. Doctors and other people in the know feel that the child shouldn't have control of daily diabetes management, Until the child clearly understands how his lifestyle, eating, exercise, rest, insulin, emotional state etc. affects his blood glucose and diabetes. If he can calculate the amount (dose) and type of insulin correctly. He's ready to assume more responsibility of his diabetes.

Future of T1DM

In near future complete cure of type 1 diabetes will be available. There is extensive research ongoing to create an oral and intranasal insulin. Soon we will have oral or nasal spray insulin. The painful injection will not be needed anymore.

Stem cell is another latest treatment. Type 1 diabetes patient gets an infusion of stem cells which helps pancreas to regenerate and produce insulin.

Other drugs such as pdx1 are being developed. It's a protein. It will help to regenerate beta cells of the pancreas.

To stop the destruction of beta cells, new drugs are being developed. The goal is to prevent T cells from killing beta cells of the pancreas.

This is an exciting time. All new drugs and treatment options are in human trail. In a few years' scientists hope to cure type 1 diabetes.

About Author

Dr. Shahriar Mostafa earned his MBBS degree in 2009. Then completed his Master's degree in Public Health in 2013. He has been working in a Medical College Hospital for last 7 years. He wants to write simple, easy to read and small patient education books to reach a larger audience.

Other Books by Dr. Shahriar

Pregnancy & Diabetes: Smallest Book with Everything You Need to Know

http://www.amazon.co.uk/gp/product/B01CEDAH08

This book gives you a complete picture on GDM (Gestational Diabetes mellitus). It also gives information on pregnancy with type 1 or type 2 diabetes. If you are a pregnant mother with or without diabetes this book gives all the information you need to protect you and your baby from the complications of GDM or other types of Diabetes.

Diagnosed with Diabetes. Now What!

https://www.amazon.com/dp/B01HC0CF26

You were living your life to the fullest. Working hard and playing harder. Ignoring symptoms like fatigue, weight loss and increased frequency of urine. Then BAM! Out of the blue you started feeling very sick. You consult with your doctor, he run some tests and you are diagnosed with diabetes! Now What!

Type 2 Diabetes: Smallest book with everything you need to know

https://www.amazon.com/dp/B01FUGZASK

Diabetes is a common disease. About 350 million people worldwide have diabetes. It is easy to control. It does not keep you from anything the life has to offer. But there is a catch, you have to control Diabetes all your life.

CPSIA information can be obtained
at www.ICGtesting.com
Printed in the USA
LVOW03s1920080517
533723LV00012B/1802/P

9 781523 675784